0 Carb, 0 Stress

40 No Carb Recipes - A Diet Book for Losing Weight; Appetizers, Sides, Sauces & Mains to Keep You Lean!

BY

Anthony Boundy

Table of Contents

INTRODUCTION 5

Appetizers, Sides, and Sauces...7

    Alfredo Sauce...8

    Avocado Butter 10

    Buffalo Chicken Egg Mayo Salad 12

    Burger Buns 14

    Cheesy Egg Fries 16

    Crab Dip..18

    Egg and Bacon Salad 20

    Homemade Blender Mayo 22

    Lemon Spinach 'Parm.'..24

    Salmon Chowder..26

Mains 28

    Baby Back Ribs..29

    Bacon and Chicken Omelette..31

    Baked Parmesan Haddock 33

    BBQ Frankfurters...35

    Beef Kebabs 37

Blackened Cajun Chicken..39

Cheesy Bacon and Sausage Breakfast Casserole..................41

Chicken with Creamy Tarragon Sauce 43

Cordon Bleu Chicken...45

Crab Cakes with Dijon Mustard..47

Grilled Crab Legs with Butter...49

Cream Cheese Pancakes 51

Deep South Chicken 53

Dijon Chicken 55

Egg and Sausage Muffins 57

Glazed Maple-Mustard Salmon 59

Goat's Cheese Omelet...61

Grilled Rosemary Swordfish...63

Indian Apricot Chicken...65

Juicy Ribeye Steak with Avocado Butter 67

Mediterranean Lemon Chicken...69

Mexican Steak Omelette 71

One-Pot Corned Beef..73

Perfect Pizza..75

Roasted Chicken 77

Sesame Ginger Pork...79

Smoky BBQ Pork Chops 81

Spicy Chicken Tenders 83

Teriyaki Pork 85

Turkey Meatballs 87

INTRODUCTION

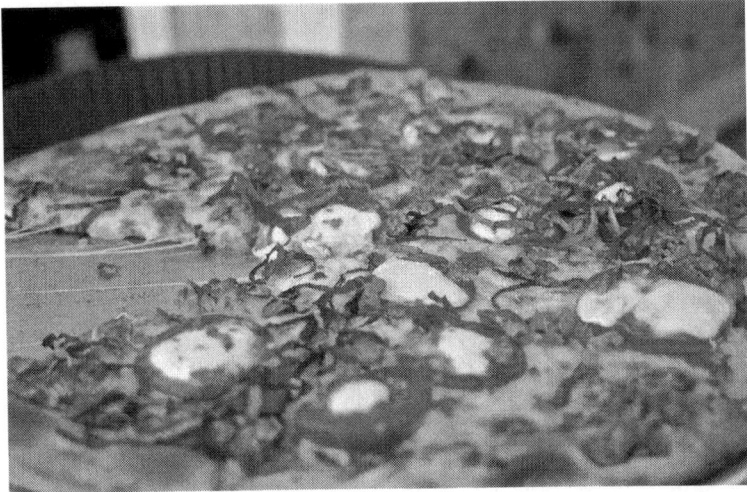

Recipes claiming to be up to 100% carb free can sometimes be a little misleading.

A number of foods including cream, fish and even seasonings and spices such as cumin, oregano, and garlic contain carbs. But use these sparingly, keep to the serving sizes in this book, and you will only be consuming trace amounts of carbs.

In some cases, if you want to eliminate these from your dietary intake altogether, you can simply take out the offending ingredient before serving. Taking advantage of the taste but still following a no carb diet plan.

A number of the recipes included in 0 Carb, 0 Stress! Use salad dressings, barbecue sauces, and sweet fruity spreads. Don't worry; all of these ingredients can be found with zero carbs in lots of health stores or online. They taste really good and are ideal for adding flavor.

It is possible to eat a varied diet and devise meal plans that will satisfy your appetite and your taste buds while avoiding carbs altogether.

Appetizers, Sides, and Sauces

Alfredo Sauce

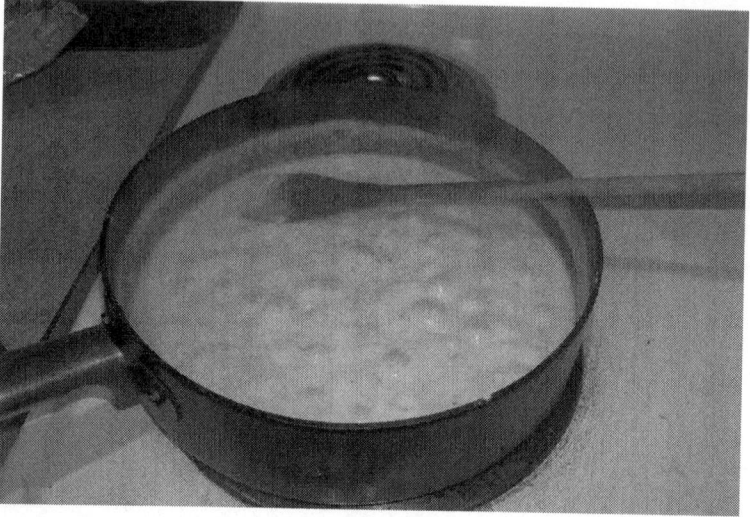

This creamy and indulgent Italian sauce is perfect for drizzling over vegetables or meat for a comforting midweek dinner.

Portions: 6-8

Prep Time: 2mins

Total Time: 12mins

Ingredients:

- 2 tbsp. of unsalted butter
- 1½ cups of heavy cream
- ½ cup of grated Parmesan

- 4 ounces of grated Romano cheese
- Pinch of black pepper
- ⅛ tsp of ground nutmeg

Directions:

1. Place a saucepan over med-high heat and melt the butter. Pour in the cream and bring to a gentle simmer for 8-9 minutes.

2. Take off the heat and sprinkle with the cheese, black pepper, and ground nutmeg. Stir well until the cheese has melted and you have a smooth sauce. Serve straight away.

Avocado Butter

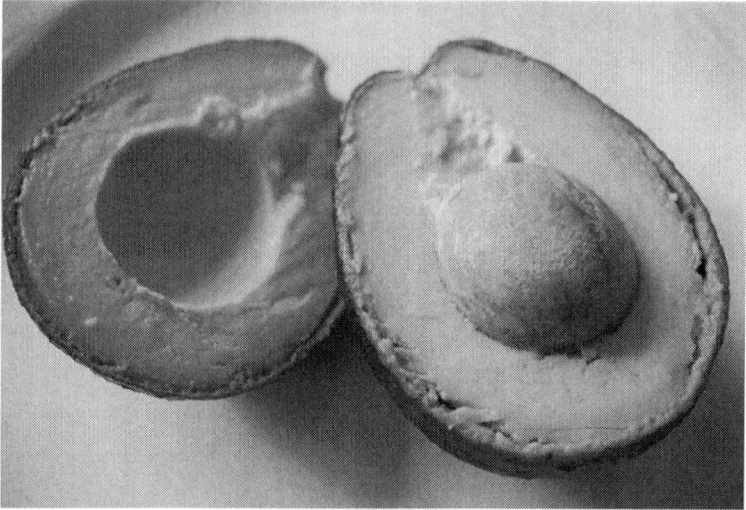

This delicious creamy butter can be made ahead and refrigerated. It makes a delicious accompaniment to grilled chicken, steak or fish.

Portions: 12-14

Prep Time: 5mins

Total Time: 4hours 5mins

Ingredients:

- 2 small avocados (stones remove and 'meat' set aside)
- 1 tbsp. of freshly squeezed lemon juice

- 2 ounces of butter (room temp)
- 1 clove of garlic (minced)
- 1 tbsp. of fresh cilantro (finely chopped)
- 2 tbsp. of cumin
- Sea salt and black pepper

Directions:

1. Add all 7 ingredients into a blender/ food processor and blitz until totally smooth. Transfer to a bowl, cover and refrigerate for 3-4 hours. When ready to serve, whip the butter a little with a fork.

Buffalo Chicken Egg Mayo Salad

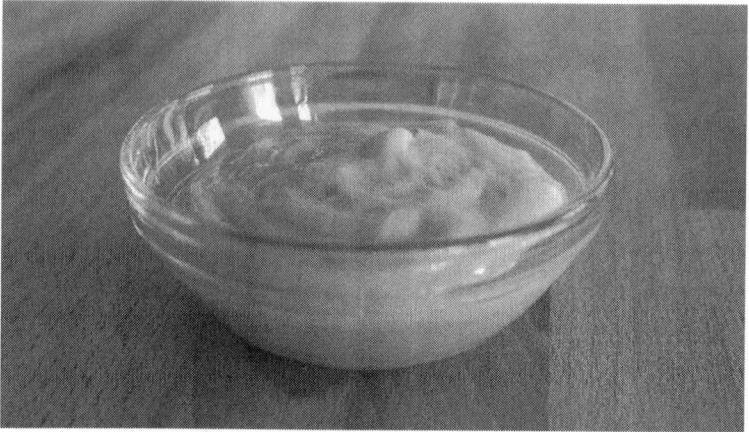

A great side dish to serve at your next cookout. Family and friends will never guess it's virtually zero carbs!

Portions: 4

Prep Time: 20mins

Total Time: 30mins

Ingredients:

- 3 hardboiled eggs (diced)
- 3 ounces of boneless cooked chicken thigh
- 1½ tbsp. of homemade mayo*
- ¾ tbsp. of hot buffalo wing sauce
- ⅛ cup of blue cheese (crumbled)

Directions:

1. Combine all ingredients in a serving bowl and toss/stir until well combined. Serve immediately or refrigerate until needed.

*Recipe for homemade mayo included in the book.

Burger Buns

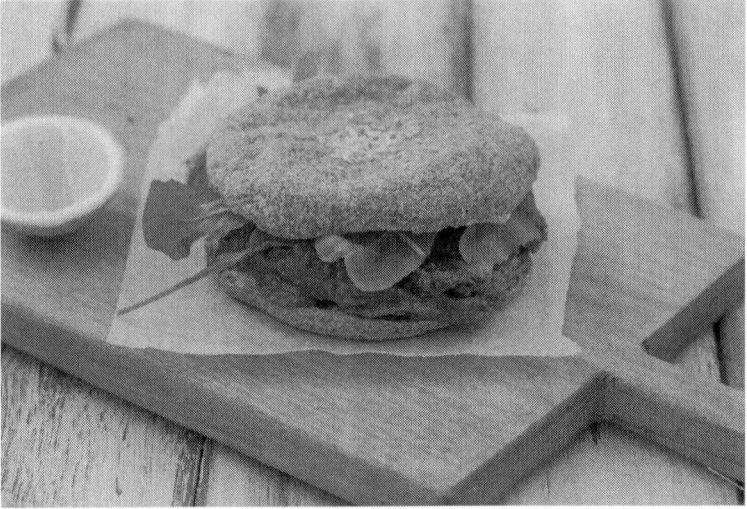

The world is now your oyster. You can enjoy a host of different fillings in your very own, carb-free bun.

Portions: 5

Prep Time: 20mins

Total Time: 40mins

Ingredients:

- 3 large eggs (separated)
- 3 tbsp. of low-fat cottage cheese
- 2 tsp of Stevia granulated sugar substitute
- ¼ tsp of cream of tartar

- Fat-free cooking spray

Directions:

1. Preheat the main oven to 350 degrees F.

2. Take the eggs and separate the white from the yolks. There must be no trace of yolk left in the white.

3. In a mixing bowl, combine the egg yolks, low-fat cottage cheese, and sugar substitute.

4. In a large bowl, add the egg whites to the cream of tartar and using an electric mixer, whisk the mixture until fluffy and light. The mixture needs to be stiff.

5. Gradually fold the yolk mixture into the egg white, using a spatula. Mix thoroughly. Do not over mix.

6. Using cooking spray, lightly coat two cookie sheets. Using a spoon, scoop up the mixture into ten circles of equal size and place on the cookie sheets. Aim for each circle is not more than ¾" thick.

7. Transfer the sheets to the center rack of the preheated oven and bake for 17-20 minutes, or until they are golden in color.

8. Remove from oven and allow to cool on a wire rack.

Cheesy Egg Fries

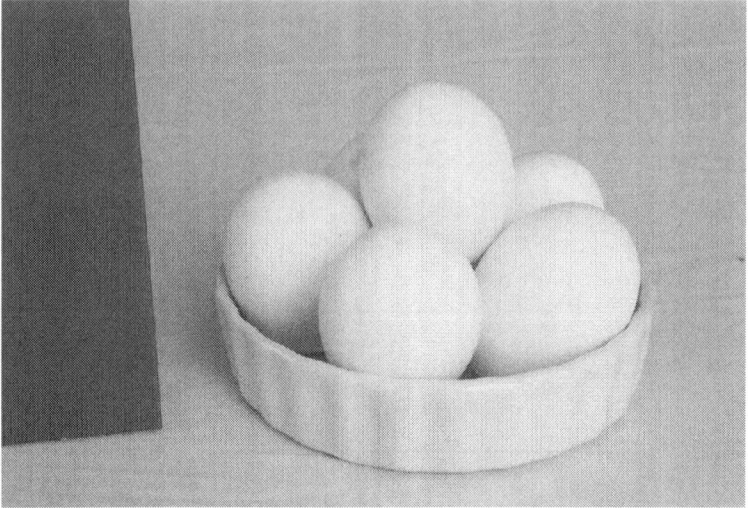

Cheesy fries, serve as a snack or with your zero-carb dip of choice.

Portions: 1

Prep Time: 2mins

Total Time: 17mins

Ingredients:

- 4 egg whites
- ½ tbsp. of cold water
- Salt
- Black Pepper

- 2 tbsp. of cheese of choice (shredded)

Directions:

1. Preheat the main oven to 400 degrees F.

2. In a medium sized bowl, whisk the egg white, cold water, salt and black pepper.

3. In a nonstick muffin pan, using a food syringe; fill each cup with an approximately ½ teaspoon of the egg mixture.

4. Sprinkle a pinch of shredded cheese onto each egg mixture. Transfer the muffin tin to the preheated oven and bake for 12-15 minutes until the mixture is crunchy. Check every few minutes as you don't want the mixture to burn.

5. Remove when cooked.

Crab Dip

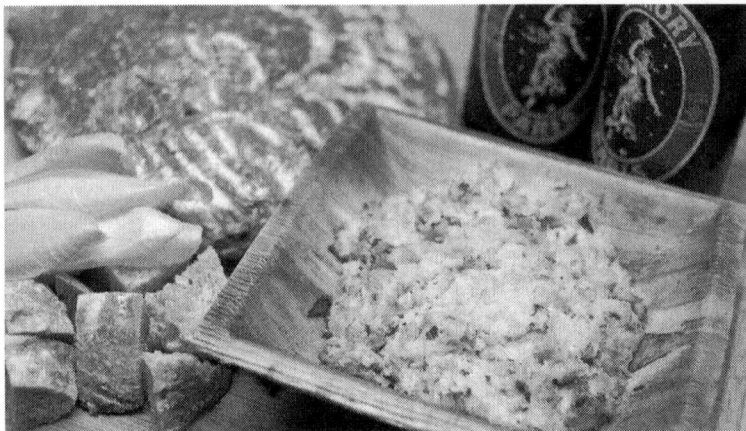

Crab meat is super healthy, high in protein, low in fat, and very, very tasty.

Portions: 4

Prep Time: 3mins

Total Time: 3mins

Ingredients:

- 1 pound of crabmeat (cooked, flaked)
- Mayonnaise
- Fish seasoning

Directions:

1. Add the crab meat into a medium bowl. Gradually add mayonnaise and seasoning to taste. Cover and chill in the refrigerator until needed.

Egg and Bacon Salad

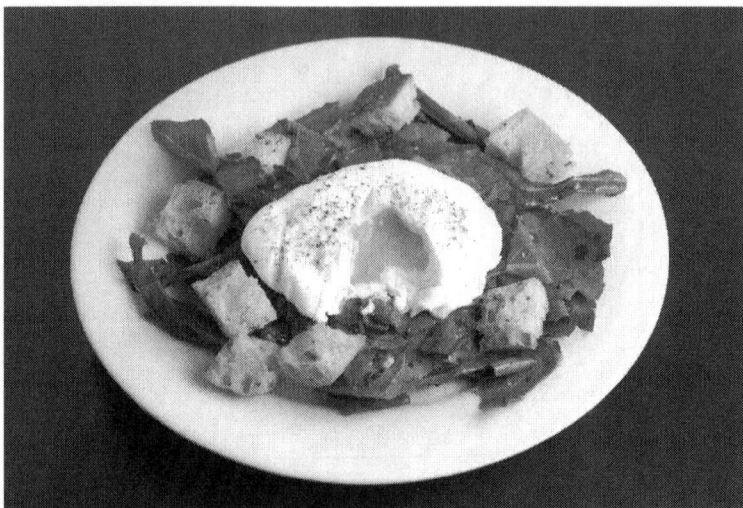

Two ingredients that go well together, so why not enjoy them as a salad? Great as an appetizer or a light bite.

Portions: 6-8

Prep Time: 10mins

Total Time: 4hours 10mins

Ingredients:

- 12 eggs (hard boiled, chopped)
- 8 rashers bacon (cooked, crumbled)
- ½ cup of crushed pork rinds
- ½ cup of mayonnaise

- Salt
- Black pepper

Directions:

1. In a large mixing bowl combine all of the ingredients and stir to combine well. Cover the bowl and place in the refrigerator to chill for 3-4 hours.

Homemade Blender Mayo

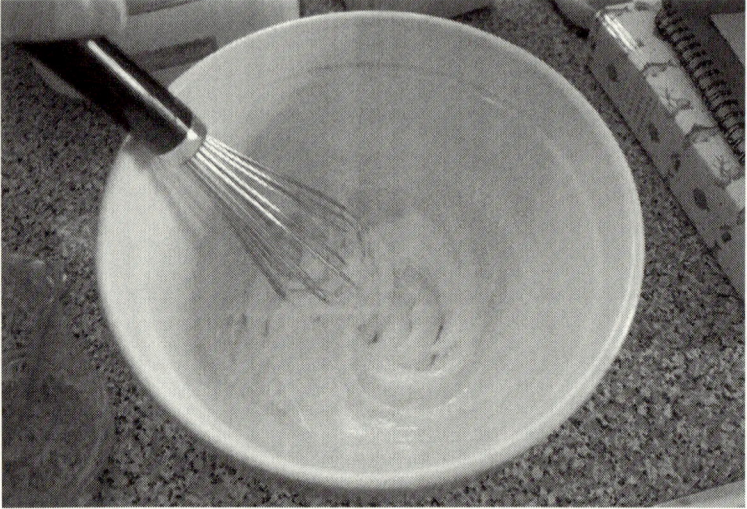

This recipe makes it simpler than ever to whip up your own mayo, free from sugar or preservatives.

Portions: 4

Prep Time: 5mins

Total Time: 5mins

Ingredients:

- 1 egg yolk
- 2 tsp of fresh squeezed lemon juice
- 1 tsp of Dijon mustard
- ½ tsp of sea salt

- Pinch of black pepper
- ½ cup of olive oil

Directions:

1. Into a blender, add the yolk, lemon juice, Dijon mustard, sea salt and black pepper. Pulse until well combined.

2. Slowly and evenly pour the oil into the blender, while on low speed until combined. Refrigerate until ready to use.

Lemon Spinach 'Parm.'

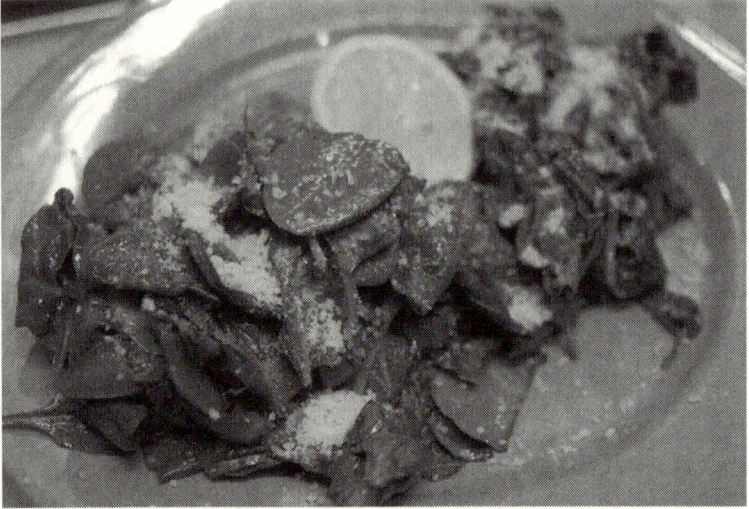

Spinach; packed with vitamins and minerals, jazz it up with fresh lemon and plenty of Parmesan!

Portions: 3-4

Prep Time: 5mins

Total Time: 1hour 25mins

Ingredients:

- 1 box of frozen spinach (thawed)
- ½ fresh lemon
- Salt and pepper (to taste)
- 1½ ounces of heavy cream

- Parmesan cheese

Directions:

1. Preheat main oven to 450 degrees F.

2. Arrange the spinach on a baking sheet, squeeze over half a fresh lemon and season with salt and pepper.

3. Roast for 8-9 minutes.

4. Transfer the roasted spinach into a saucepan, pour in the heavy cream and grate over a generous amount of Parmesan. Sauté for 3-4 minutes until heated through. Transfer to a square baking dish and allow to cool and set before slicing and digging in.

Salmon Chowder

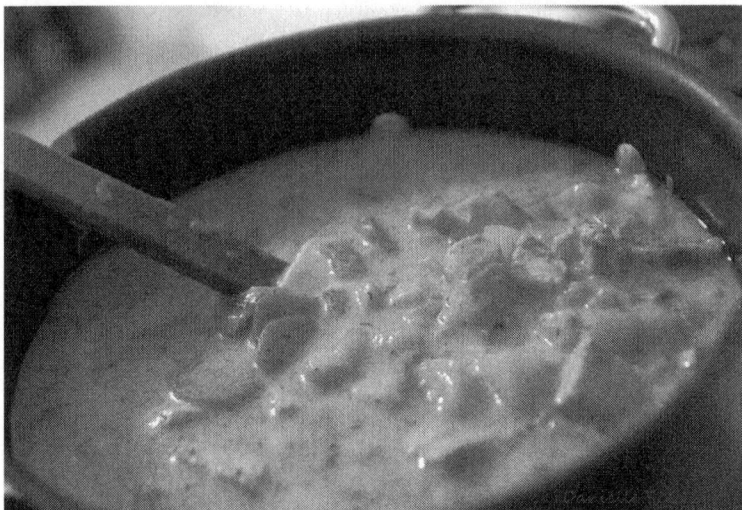

This chowder is excellent served in soup cups. It is rich and creamy, and a little does go a long way.

Portions: 2-4

Prep Time: 5mins

Total Time: 30mins

Ingredients:

- Butter (for frying)
- ½ pound of bacon (cut into ½ cubes)
- 2 pounds of salmon
- Dill

- Chives
- Salt
- Black pepper
- 16 ounces of clam broth
- 8 ounces of heavy cream

Directions:

1. Heat a large pot over medium heat and melt the butter. Add the bacon to the pot, stirring occasionally, fry until crisp and brown.

2. While the bacon is cooking, roughly chop the salmon into pieces.

3. Scatter the bacon with a little dill, chives, salt and black pepper. Next, add the salmon pieces to the pot. Stir a little and allow the fish to fry in the grease from the bacon for 1-2 minutes. Stir a couple of times.

4. Add the clam broth. Increase the heat and allow the chowder to come to a simmer. Once simmering, immediately reduce the heat back to medium-low. Continue to simmer for around 8-10 minutes.

5. When the salmon is sufficiently cooked, add a pinch of salt and pepper more. Add more dill and chives if required. Gradually pour in the heavy cream, tasting it as you do.

6. When you are happy with the seasonings, return to simmer for a couple of minutes and serve.

Mains

Baby Back Ribs

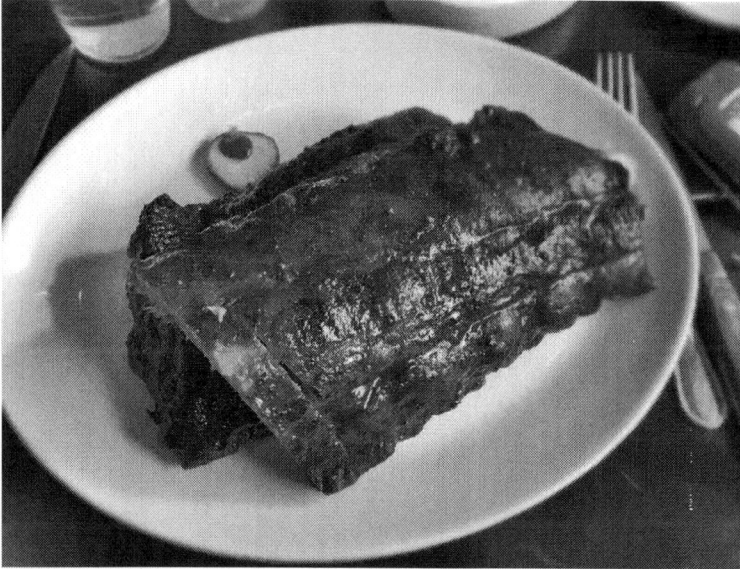

Smoky, sweet ribs slowly cooked on the barbecue. An ideal dish for a summer cookout.

Portions: 2

Prep Time: 20mins

Total Time: 15hours

Ingredients:

- 1 whole rack baby back ribs
- 1 bottle of Zero Carb BBQ sauce (any brand)
- 2 tbsp. of sugar substitute (e.g. stevia)

- ½ cup of cider vinegar
- ¼ cup of soy sauce
- Black pepper

Directions:

1. Slice the rack into 4 pieces and place them all in an extra-large resealable zipped food bag.

2. In a food blender of choice, add the remaining 5 ingredients and blitz until smooth. Add the mixture to the bag of ribs. Gently massage the bag, ensuring that all the ribs are all covered with the marinade. Transfer the bag to the refrigerator and allow to marinate overnight. Turn the bag once or twice to ensure full coverage.

3. Take the ribs out of the bag and retain the marinade for basting. On a barbecue grill cook the ribs for approximately 3-4 hours, basting with the marinade several times throughout the cooking process.

4. Remove from grill and enjoy hot.

Bacon and Chicken Omelette

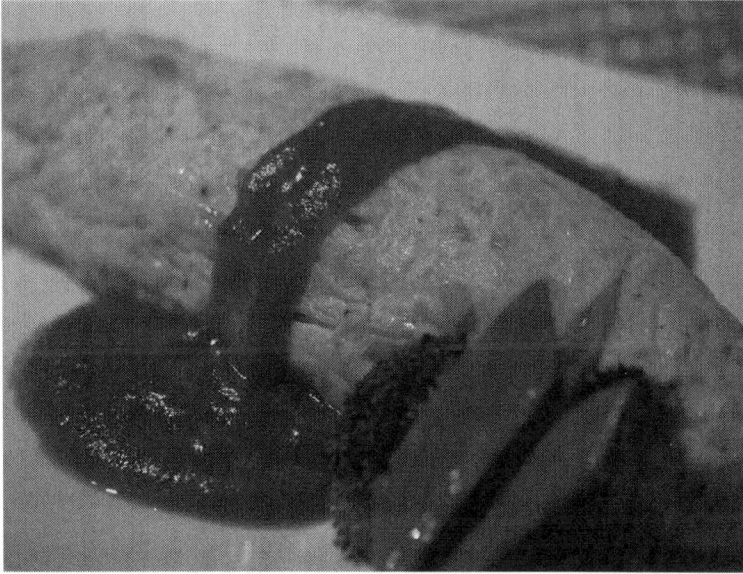

Chicken and bacon marry well together to form the perfect omelette.

Portions: 1

Prep Time: 2mins

Total Time: 10mins

Ingredients:

- 3 large eggs
- 2 tbsp. of heavy cream
- Salt

- Black pepper
- 1 tbsp. of butter
- 2 bacon slices (crumbled)
- ¼ cup of chicken (cooked, chopped)

Directions:

1. In a medium mixing bowl, beat the eggs, heavy cream, salt, and black pepper. In an omelet pan, heat the butter over a medium heat and add the egg-cream mixture. Gently lift the edges of the omelet as it cooks to prevent it from sticking to the pan.

2. When the omelet is cooked to your desired consistency, add the cooked bacon and chicken. Fold the omelet over.

3. Serve right away.

Baked Parmesan Haddock

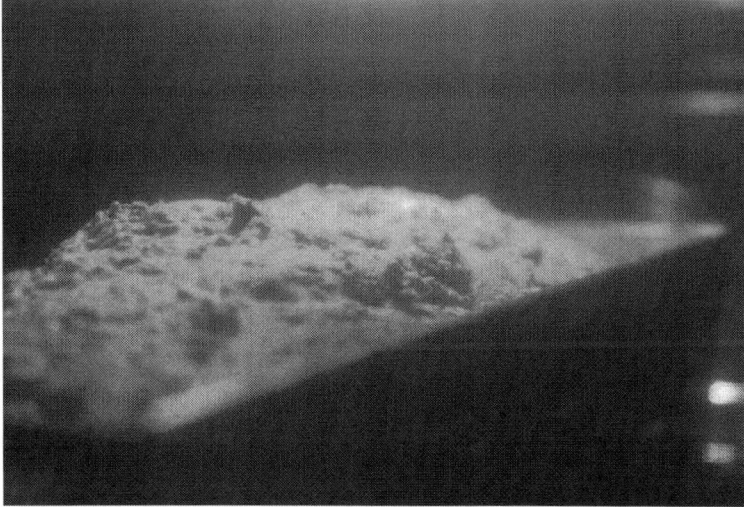

You can substitute haddock with either catfish or flounder.
If you don't mind, add 1 carb to the meal, a clove of minced
garlic to the butter.

Portions: 4

Prep Time: 2mins

Total Time: 12mins

Ingredients:

- ¼ cup of butter (melted)
- 4 haddock fillets
- Salt

- Black pepper
- Parmesan cheese (zero carbs, grated)

Directions:

1. Preheat the main oven to 425 degrees F.

2. Add the butter to a large roasting pan. Season the haddock filets with salt, and black pepper. Scatter the Parmesan on top of each fillet.

3. Cook in the preheated oven for 8-10 minutes.

BBQ Frankfurters

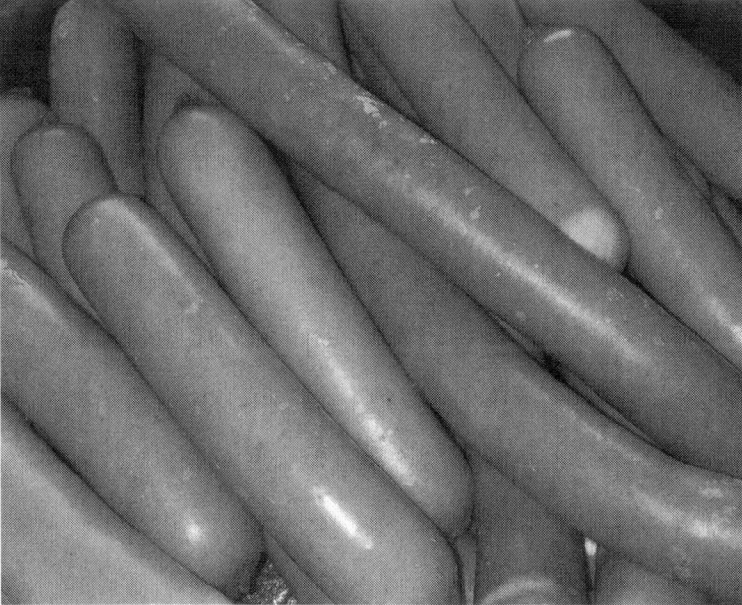

A quick and easy snack or light lunch; ideal for the weekend.

Portions: 4-6

Prep Time: 3mins

Total Time: 18mins

Ingredients:

- 2 tbsp. of vegetable oil
- 1 pack of frankfurters (zero carbs, sliced)

- 1 jar of hickory smoked BBQ sauce (zero carbs)
- 1 tbsp. of vinegar
- Brown sugar (zero carbs)

Directions:

1. In a large frying pan, heat the vegetable oil over medium heat. Brown the sliced frankfurters on both sides. Add the remaining 3 ingredients to the pan. Bring to boiling point. Cover the pan and allow to simmer for between 12-15 minutes.

2. Enjoy!

Beef Kebabs

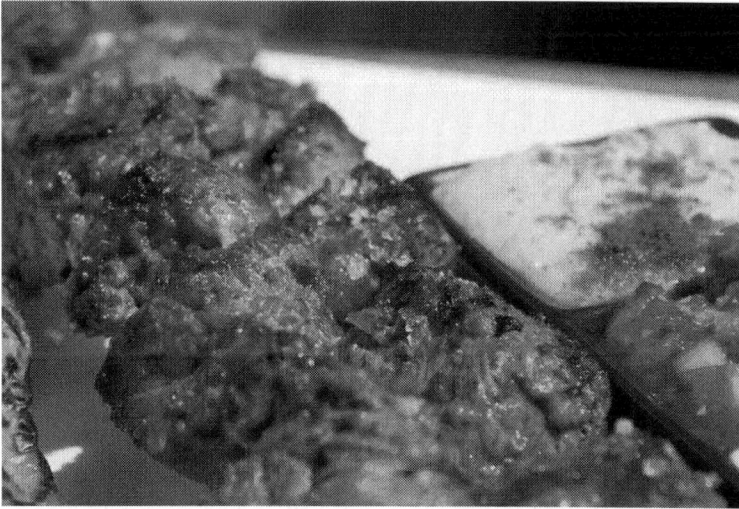

Tender kebabs marinated overnight for maximum flavor.

Portions: 6

Prep Time: 10mins

Total Time: 8hours 25mins

Ingredients:

- 2 pounds of sirloin steak (cubed)
- ¾ cup of vegetable oil
- ½ cup of soy sauce (zero carbs)
- 1 tbsp. of dry mustard
- 1-2 tsp of lemon extract

- Salt
- Black pepper
- 6 metal skewers

Directions:

1. To a shallow dish, add the cubed steak. Add the remaining 6 food ingredients to a food blender and blitz until smooth. Pour the mixture over the beef steak, cover with aluminum foil and place in the refrigerator overnight. Turn the meat over a few times during the time it is marinating.

2. Preheat the grill to a medium heat setting. String the beef cubes onto metal skewers and grill for between 12-15 minutes, continually turning.

Blackened Cajun Chicken

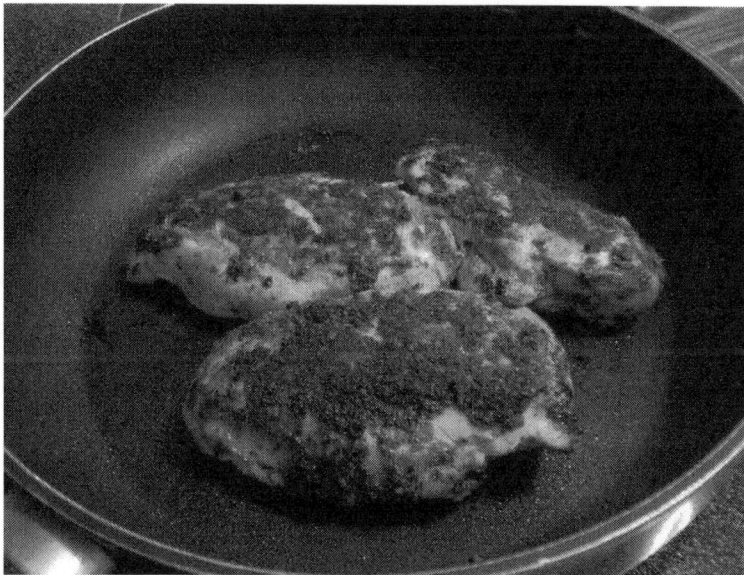

Succulent chicken served on the bone with a spicy Cajun kick. Delicious!

Portions: 4

Prep Time: 10mins

Total Time: 55mins

Ingredients:

- 4 chicken breasts (on bone with skin)
- 2 tbsp. of olive oil
- 2 tbsp. of blackened Cajun seasoning

Ingredients:

1. Preheat the grill to high heat.

2. Generously brush the chicken breasts with olive oil. Season well with Cajun seasoning and rub the seasoning all over the skin.

3. Grill the chicken for 40-45 minutes, or until the juice run clear, and the skin is crispy.

4. Enjoy!

Cheesy Bacon and Sausage Breakfast Casserole

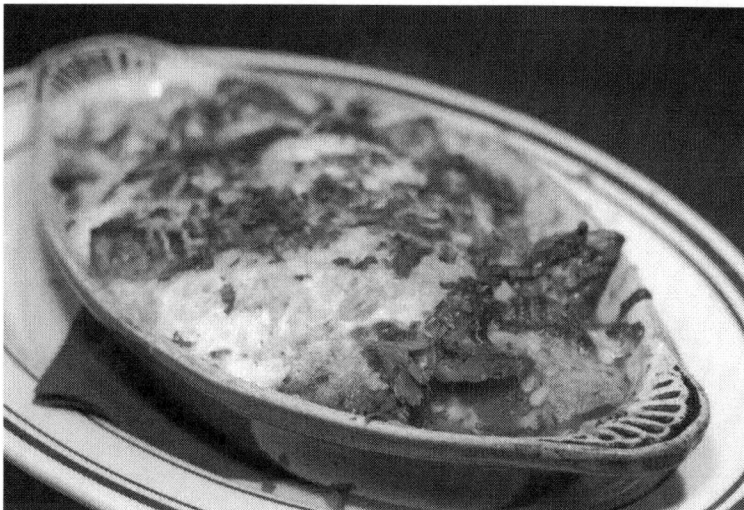

A hearty breakfast or great evening meal. Enjoy this tasty, versatile casserole any time of the day.

Portions: 12

Prep Time: 15mins

Total Time: 1hour 25mins

Ingredients:

- 1 pound of bacon (crisp, crumbled)
- 1 pound of zero carb sausage (browned)

- 12 medium eggs (beaten)
- ¼ cup of heavy whipping cream
- 2 cups of cheddar cheese (zero carbs, shredded)
- Salt and pepper

Directions:

1. Preheat the main oven to 375 degrees F.

2. Cook the bacon until crisp and the sausage until browned; drain any excess fat.

3. In a large, butter greased casserole or pie dish combine the bacon with the sausage.

4. In a medium sized mixing bowl, beat the eggs and cream until combined. Add the cheddar cheese and season well with salt and black pepper.

5. Transfer the mixture to the greased dish and bake for 50-60 minutes.

Chicken with Creamy Tarragon Sauce

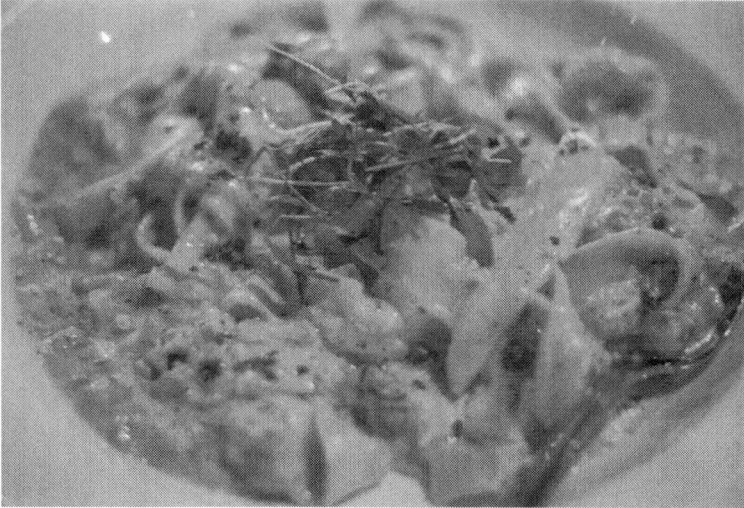

Nothing beats a good hunk of steak, especially when topped with a dollop of creamy avocado butter.

Portions: 4

Prep Time: 5mins

Total Time: 25mins

Ingredients:

- 1 tbsp. of unsalted butter
- 1 tbsp. of canola oil
- 32 ounces of boneless chicken breasts
- ½ cup of heavy cream

- 1 tbsp. of Dijon mustard
- ¾ tsp of tarragon
- Sea salt and black pepper (to taste)

Directions:

1. Melt together the butter and oil in a large skillet. Brown the chicken on both sides. Turn down the heat and cook for 15 minutes.

2. Remove the chicken from the skillet and set aside (covered).

3. Pour the cream into the skillet to deglaze. Add in the Dijon and tarragon. Cook until the sauce thickens (4-5 minutes).

4. Season with salt and pepper and stir.

5. Pour the sauce over the chicken and serve immediately.

Cordon Bleu Chicken

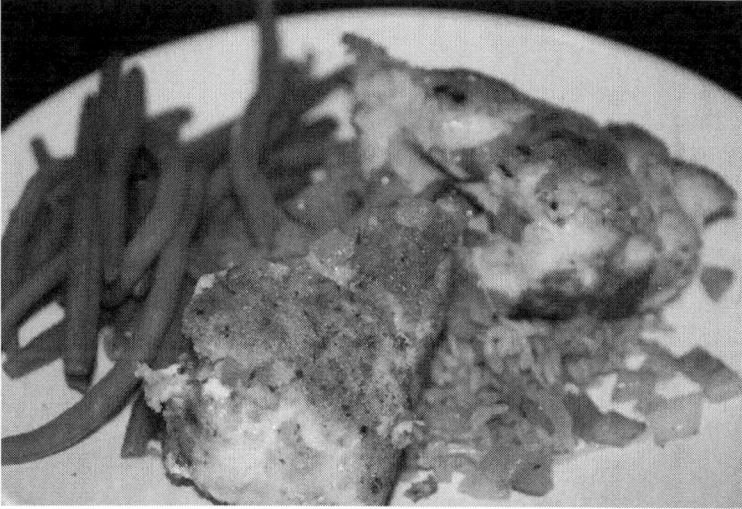

Friends and family will be amazed that this chicken dish has zero carbs. An excellent mid -week meal.

Portions: 4

Prep Time: 10mins

Total Time: 1hour 10mins

Ingredients:

- 4 chicken breasts (boneless, skinless)
- Salt
- Black pepper
- 4 slices of cooked ham

- 4 slices of Swiss cheese (zero carbs)
- ½ cup of crushed pork rinds

Directions:

1. Preheat the main oven to 350 degrees F.

2. Using a mallet pound each of the chicken breasts to no more than a ¼" thick. Season each piece of chicken with salt and black pepper. Place one slice of ham and one slice of cheese on top of each chicken piece. Roll each piece and secure with a cocktail stick.

3. Transfer each roll to a baking tin and scatter with crushed pork rinds.

4. Cook in the preheated oven for between 45-60 minutes.

Crab Cakes with Dijon Mustard

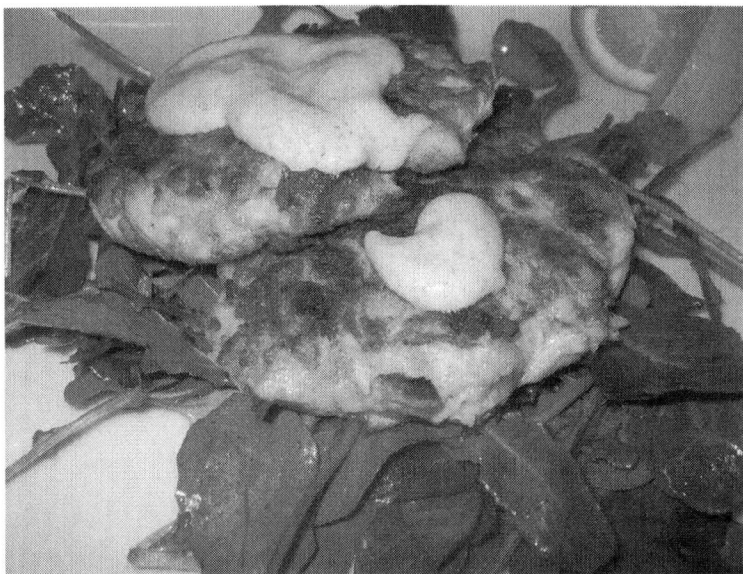

The sweet crab combines with the hot spicy Dijon mustard to deliver a pattie that no-one can resist.

Portions: 4

Prep Time: 5mins

Total Time: 15mins

Ingredients:

- 1 pound of lump crab
- 1 tbsp. of Dijon mustard
- 2 tbsp. of mayonnaise

- 2 egg yolks (beaten)
- 1 cup of crushed pork rinds
- 4 tbsp. of butter

Directions:

1. In a large mixing bowl combine the lump crab, Dijon mustard, mayonnaise, beaten egg yolk, and crushed pork rinds. Mix thoroughly.

2. Wearing disposable gloves, form the mixture into equal sized patties. Transfer the patties to the refrigerator and chill overnight.

3. In a skillet, melt the butter over a medium heat and cook the crab cake patties for 3-5 minutes on each side, or until they are golden brown.

Grilled Crab Legs with Butter

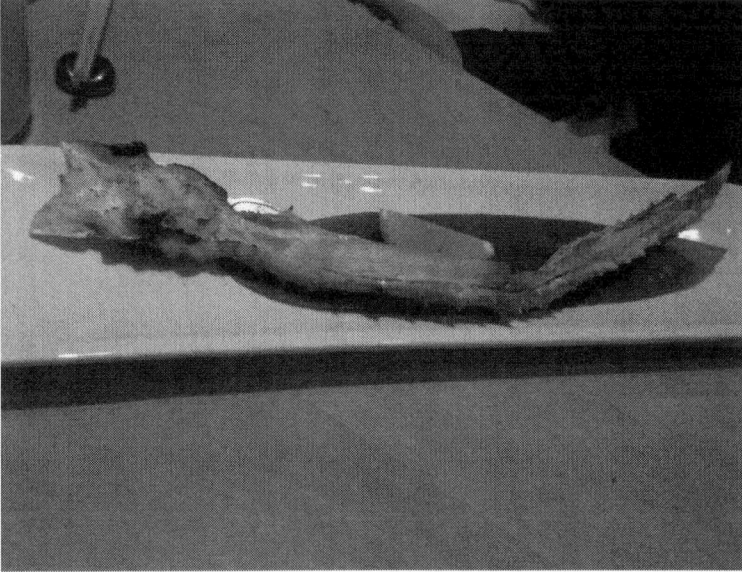

Protein packed crab legs are the way to healthy eating for everyone, even those who are not following a zero-carb regime.

Portions: 2

Prep Time: 5mins

Total Time: 30mins

Ingredients:

- 1 pound of fresh/frozen Snow Crab leg clusters (if frozen, thawed)

- ¼ cup of butter
- 1 garlic clove (minced)
- 1½ tsp of dried parsley
- ⅛ tsp of salt
- ¼ tsp of black pepper

Directions:

1. Cut a lengthwise slit into each crab shell.

2. In a large heavy frying pan or skillet, melt the butter over medium-low heat. Add the garlic and cook until the garlic emits its fragrant aroma. Stir in the dried parsley, salt, and black pepper. Simmer the butter for around 15 minutes or until it gently foams. Take care not to burn the butter.

3. Allow the butter to totally cool before skimming off the foam. Add the crab legs, tossing well in the butter mixture to coat all over. Simmer until cooked, for approx. 5-7 minutes.

4. Serve hot.

Cream Cheese Pancakes

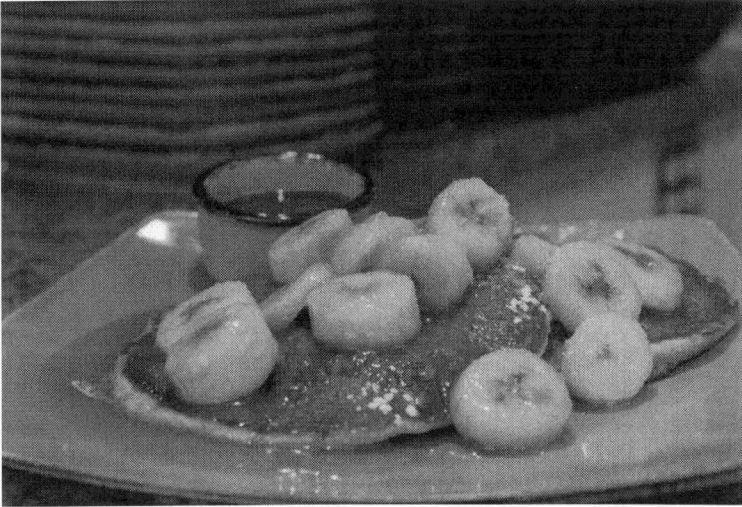

Enjoy as an appetizer, light meal or even for breakfast with a side of bacon. If you aren't a fan of cream cheese – experiment!

Portions: 4

Prep Time: 2mins

Total Time: 10mins

Ingredients:

- 2 ounces of cream cheese
- 2 eggs
- ½ tsp of cinnamon

Directions:

1. In a blender of choice, combine all the ingredients and blitz until smooth. Allow to rest for a couple of minutes to let the bubbles settle.

2. Pour ¼ of the batter mixture into a skillet, greased with butter. Cook on medium to high heat for approx. 2 minutes, or until golden brown. Flip the pancakes over and cook on the reverse side. Repeat the process until all of the pancake mixtures has been used.

3. Enjoy warm.

Deep South Chicken

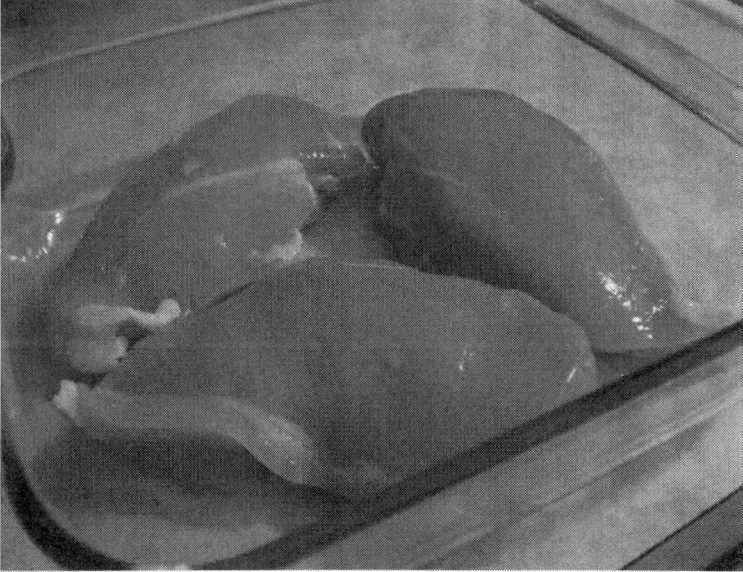

A rich tasting chicken for adults only!

Portions: 4

Prep Time: 10mins

Total Time: 10hours

Ingredients:

- 4 chicken breasts
- 1 bottle of sesame ginger dressing (zero carbs, any brand)
- ½ cup of soy sauce

- ¼ cup of brown sugar (zero carbs)
- ½ cup of bourbon
- Salt
- Black pepper

Directions:

1. Add the chicken breasts to a large, resealable zipped bag.

2. In a mixing bowl, combine the remaining 6 ingredients and stir well. Pour the mixture over the chicken in the bag. Massage the bag gently to ensure that the chicken breasts are evenly covered. Place the bag in the refrigerator overnight.

3. Preheat your main oven to 350 degrees F.

4. Pour the contents of the bag, including the marinade, into a large casserole dish and place in the oven for 1-1 ½ hours, or until the chicken's juices run clear.

Dijon Chicken

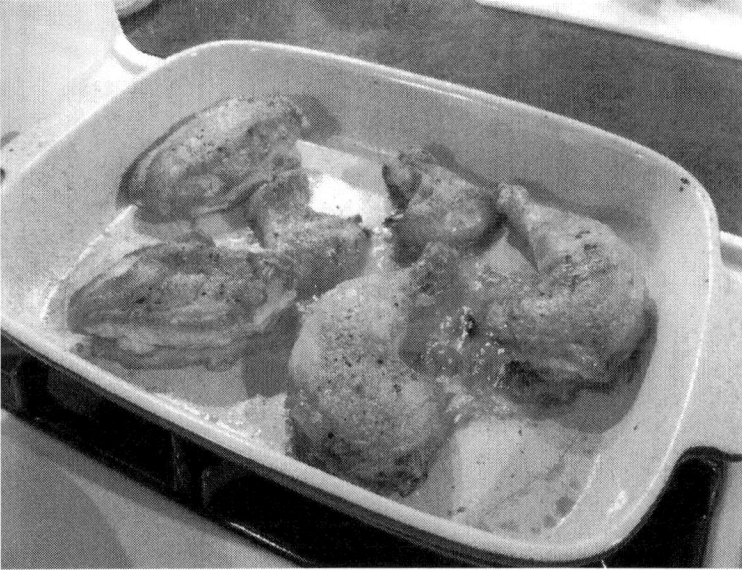

The tangy mustard sauce is the perfect accompaniment for moist, juicy chicken.

Portions: 4

Prep Time: 10mins

Total Time: 35mins

Ingredients:

- 4 boneless chicken breasts (halved)
- 4 tbsp. of olive oil
- 3 cloves of garlic (minced)

- 5 tbsp. of low sodium soy sauce
- 3 ounces of white cooking wine (non-alcoholic)
- 4 tbsp. of Dijon mustard

Directions:

1. Place each chicken breast between two pieces of cling film and using a heavy pan or mallet pound until the breasts are no more than ½" thick.

2. In a skillet, over medium heat, heat the olive oil. When hot, add the chicken, and brown on both sides.

3. Add the remaining 5 ingredients to a medium sized mixing bowl. Stir thoroughly to combine.

4. Once the chicken is golden, reduce the heat to low and pour the mustard-wine mixture over the chicken pieces. Cook in the skillet until the chicken's juices run clear.

5. Spoon a little of the Dijon mustard sauce over the chicken before serving.

Egg and Sausage Muffins

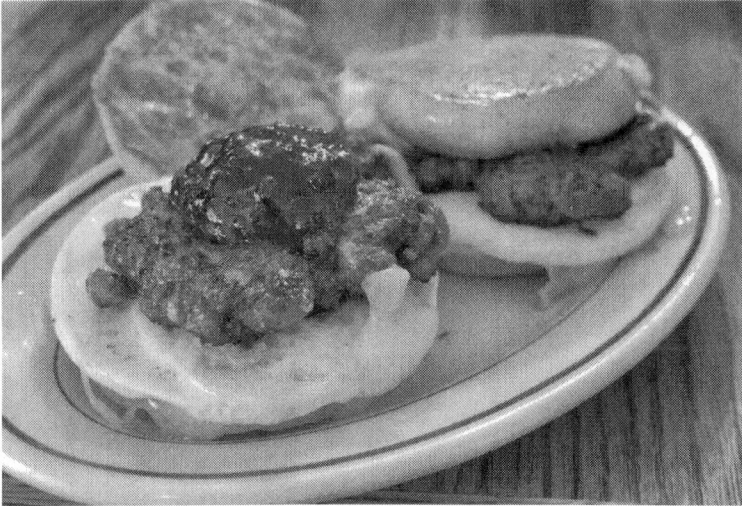

What better way to start the day than with hot, tasty breakfast muffins?

Portions: 6

Prep Time: 10mins

Total Time: 35mins

Ingredients:

- 1 tbsp. of butter
- 2 spicy Italian sausage links (cut into bite-size slices)
- 6 medium eggs

- 2 tsp of hot sauce
- Red pepper flakes
- 1 cup of cheddar cheese (shredded)
- Fresh cracked pepper

Directions:

1. Pre-heat the main oven to 350 degrees F. Using non-stick cooking spray, lightly grease an extra-large muffin tin.

2. In a skillet, over medium heat, sauté the butter and sausage link slices. Place an equal amount of sausage in each of the muffin tray cups.

3. In a medium bowl, beat the eggs, hot sauce, and pepper flakes. Add the cheddar cheese and stir to combine. Pour an even amount of the egg mixture over the sausage.

4. Bake in the center of the preheated oven for 18-20 minutes. Turn the heat off and allow the muffins to set for an additional 4-5 minutes before taking out of the oven.

Glazed Maple-Mustard Salmon

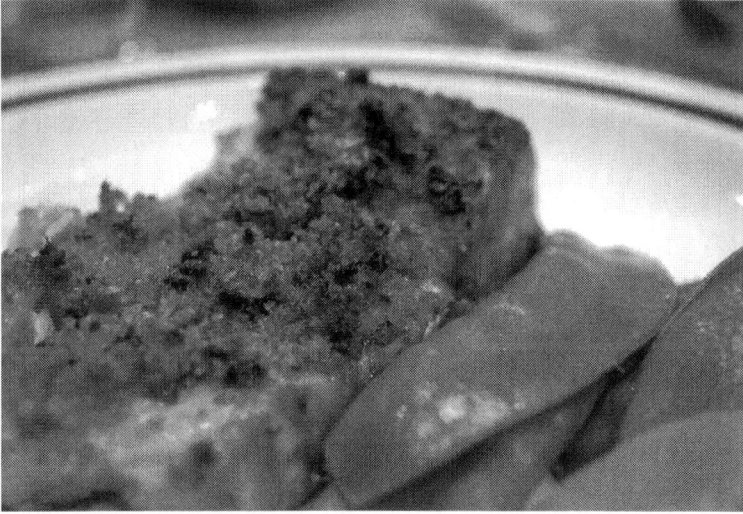

A delicious recipe that all the family will love.

Portions: 4

Prep Time: 15mins

Total Time: 25mins

Ingredients:

- ¼ cup of maple syrup (zero carbs)
- ½ cup of water
- 2 tsp of Dijon mustard
- 2 garlic cloves
- ¼ tsp of sea salt

- 2 pounds of salmon

Directions:

1. In a small or medium saucepan, add the maple syrup, water, Dijon mustard, garlic and sea salt. Bring to a simmer and leave until you see the liquid is reduced to roughly half a cup. Take off the heat and allow to cool.

2. Preheat the broiler. On an oiled rack of a broiler pan, arrange the salmon (skin down). Sprinkle with a little salt and broil for 6-8 minutes. Remove and generously brush with the maple sauce. Return to the broiler for 3-4 more minutes. Serve immediately.

Goat's Cheese Omelet

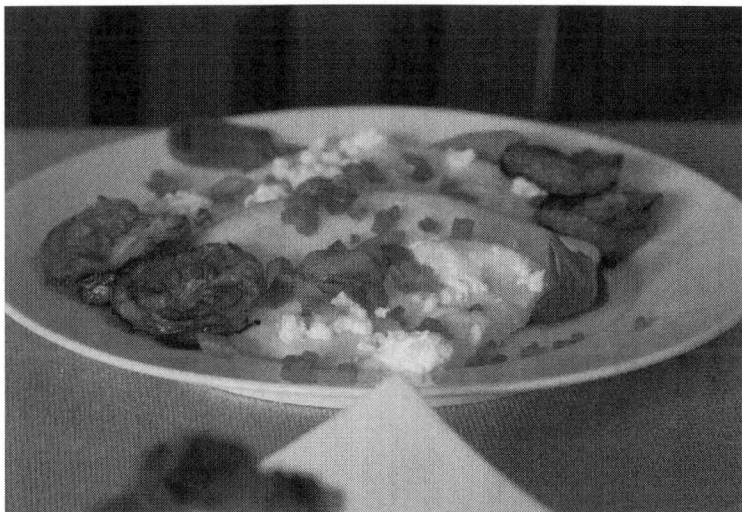

Although this works for a lot of different varieties of cheese, goat's cheese has a particularly good flavor. You could also add a teaspoon of parsley or basil to the mix.

Portions: 1

Prep Time: 3mins

Total Time: 8mins

Ingredients:

- 3 large eggs
- 2 tbsp. of heavy cream
- ½ tsp of salt

- ¼ tsp of black pepper
- 1 tbsp. of butter
- 2 ounces of goat cheese (crumbled)

Directions:

1. In a medium bowl whisk the eggs, cream, salt and black pepper.

2. In a small frying pan or skillet melt the butter. Add the whisked eggs and cook until nearly set. Add the crumbled goat cheese over the omelet and fold. Continue to cook for a minute or so, until the goat's cheese has melted.

3. Remove from pan and enjoy.

Grilled Rosemary Swordfish

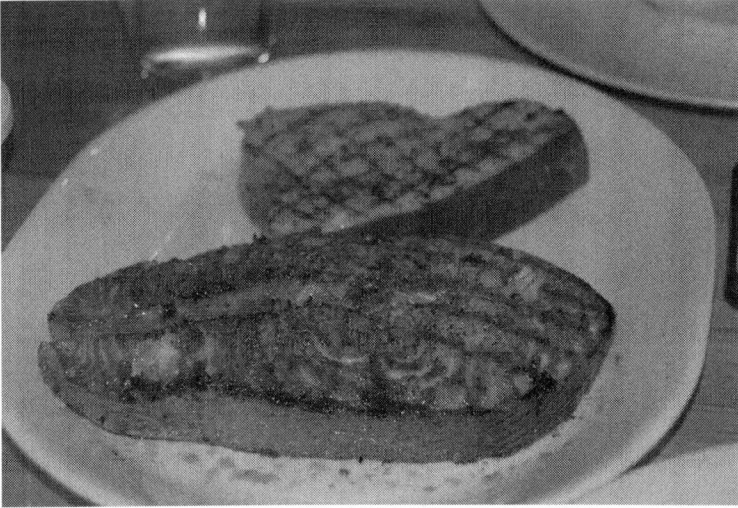

This recipe comes in at 2g of carbs per serving. If you want to be carb-free, then don't include the garlic. Alternatively, you could leave the garlic whole and discard it before serving. That way you have the flavor with the carbs.

Portions: 2

Prep Time: 10mins

Total Time: 20mins

Ingredients:

- 1 tbsp. of lemon juice
- 1 tbsp. of olive oil

- 2 garlic of cloves (minced)
- 1 tsp of fresh rosemary (minced)
- 1 tsp of lemon peel (grated)
- ¼ tsp of salt
- ¼ tsp of pepper
- 2 (5 ounces) of swordfish steaks

Directions:

1. Combine the first 7 ingredients in a zip lock bag. Add the swordfish steaks and seal the bag. Massage gently and ensure that each steak is evenly coated. Place the bag in the refrigerator for 60 minutes.

2. Drain off and discard the marinade. Using a piece of kitchen paper, moistened with cooking oil, lightly coat the grill rack. Place the swordfish on the rack, cover with aluminum foil, and over a medium to high heat cook for 4-6 on each side, or until the swordfish becomes opaque.

Indian Apricot Chicken

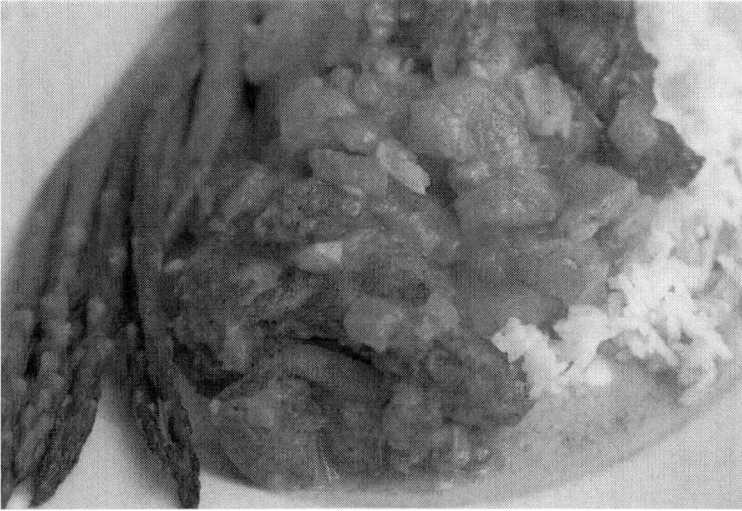

A healthy way to enjoy the exotic flavors of Indian cooking – who needs take-outs with dishes like this!

Portions: 6-8

Prep Time: 15mins

Total Time: 8hours 15mins

Ingredients:

- 1 whole chicken (cut into pieces)
- Garlic powder
- Onion powder
- Salt

- Black pepper
- 1 tbsp. of butter
- ½ cup of chicken broth
- 1 jar of apricot fruit spread (zero carbs, any brand)
- 2 tsp of garam masala
- 1 tsp of curry powder

Directions:

1. Season the cut chicken well with garlic powder, onion powder, salt and black pepper.

2. In a large frying pan or skillet, melt the butter over medium heat. Add the cut chicken to the pan and cook until golden brown. Transfer the cooked chicken to a slow cooker.

3. Use the chicken broth to deglaze your pan and pour the broth over the chicken in the slow cooker.

4. In a medium bowl, combine the remaining 4 ingredients and stir well. Pour the mixture over the chicken and set the slow cooker to low. Cook the apricot chicken for 6-8 hours.

Juicy Ribeye Steak with Avocado Butter

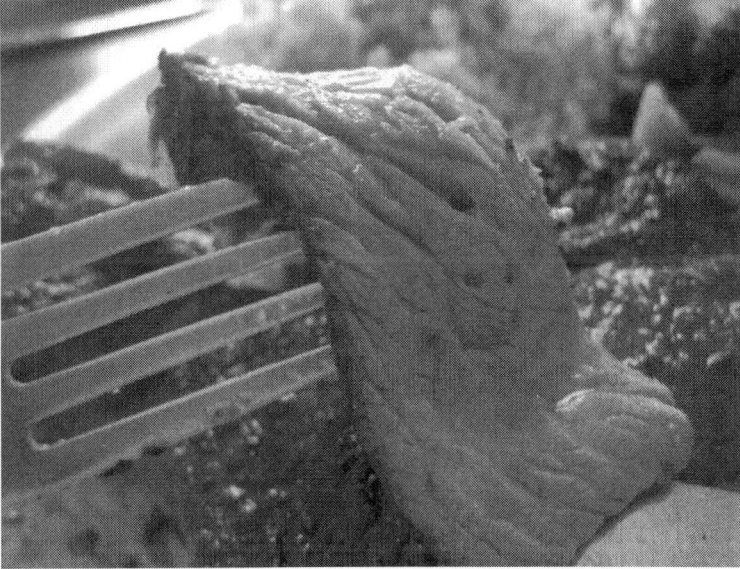

Nothing beats a good hunk of steak, especially when topped with a dollop of creamy avocado butter.

Portions: 4

Prep Time: 5mins

Total Time: 15mins

Ingredients:

- 28 ounces of rib eye steak

- ½ tsp of fresh garlic
- 1 tbsp. of parsley
- Sea salt and black pepper (to taste)
- 4 tbsp. of avocado butter*

Directions:

1. Rub all of the steaks (both sides) with the garlic and parsley, then season with salt and pepper.

2. Place the steaks on the rack of a broiler pan. Broil until medium rare (approximately 10 minutes).

3. Serve each steak immediately with a dollop of avocado butter on top.

*Recipe for avocado butter included in the book.

Mediterranean Lemon Chicken

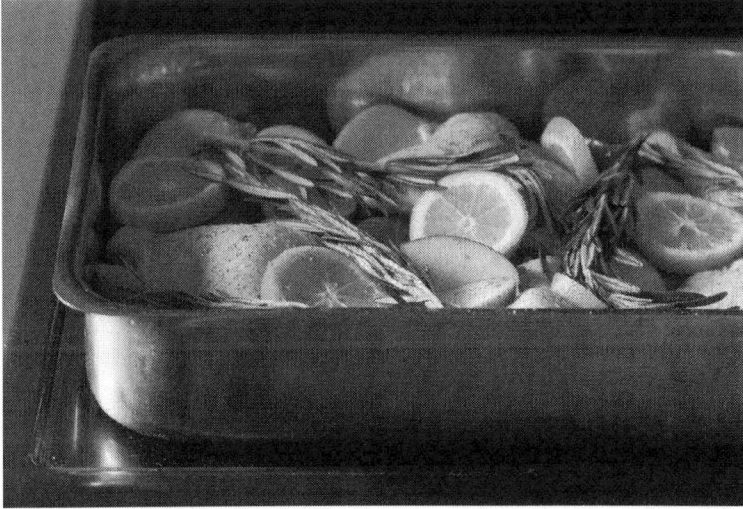

Slow cookers are the convenient way of providing healthy meals during the week.

Portions: 6

Prep Time: 10mins

Total Time: 8hours 20mins

Ingredients:

- 1 whole chicken (cut into pieces)
- Onion powder
- Garlic powder
- Salt

- Black pepper
- ¼ cup of butter
- ½ cup of chicken broth
- 3 tbsp. of lemon extract
- Pinch of dried oregano

Directions:

1. Season the cut chicken pieces with onion powder, garlic powder, salt and black pepper.

2. In a large frying pan or skillet over medium melt the butter. Add the chicken to the pan and cook until golden brown. Transfer the cooked chicken to a slow cooker.

3. Use the chicken broth to deglaze the pan and pour the broth over the chicken in the slow cooker. Sprinkle the 3 tablespoons of lemon extract and oregano on top of the chicken and cook on low heat for between 6-8 hours.

Mexican Steak Omelette

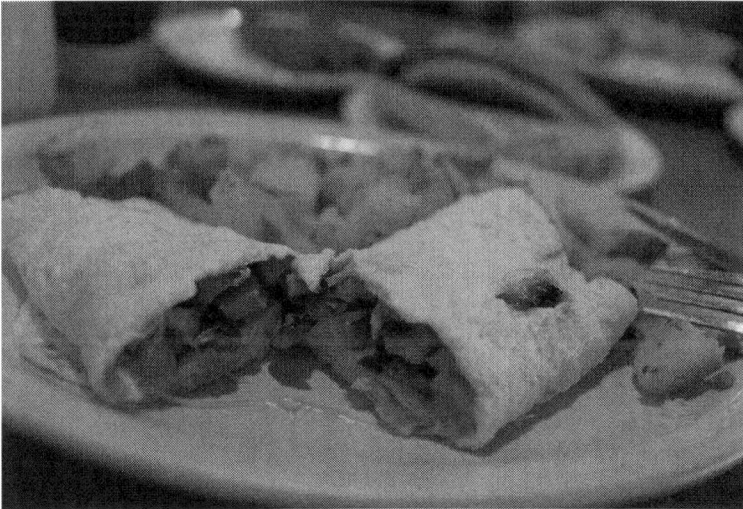

A great zero carb way to enjoy a taste of Mexico.

Portions: 1

Prep Time: 1min

Total Time: 10mins

Ingredients:

- 4 ounces of ground sirloin
- ½ tsp of taco seasoning
- 3 eggs
- 2 tbsp. of creamer (zero carbs)
- Salt

- Black pepper
- 1 tbsp. of butter
- Cheddar cheese (zero carbs, shredded)

Directions:

1. In a large skillet, over med-high heat, add the ground sirloin. Sprinkle the sirloin with the taco seasoning. Cook the meat until well browned. Set it to one side and cover to keep warm.

2. Using a medium bowl, beat together the eggs, creamer, salt and black pepper.

3. In a small frying pan, heat the butter and add the omelet mixture. As the omelet cooks, carefully lift it to allow air to flow underneath. When cooked to your satisfaction, add the cooked sirloin, sprinkle with cheddar cheese and fold over. Allow to cook for a minute or so to melt the cheese and serve.

One-Pot Corned Beef

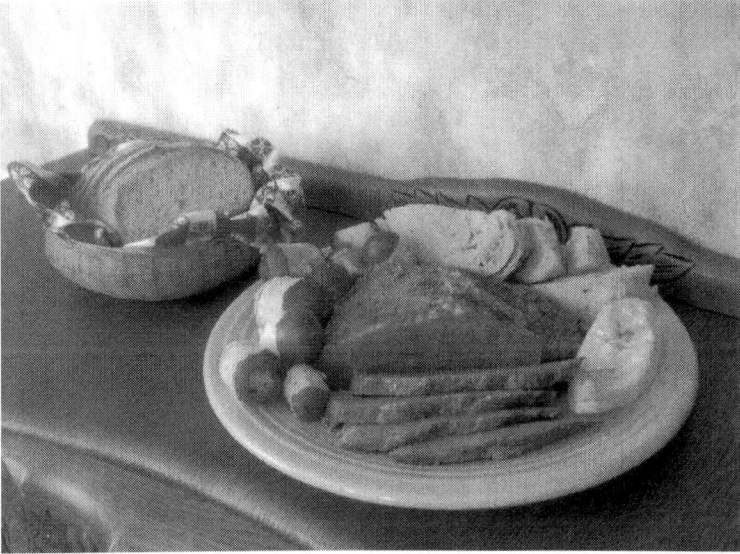

A hearty meal ideal for the weekend when all the family is together.

Portions: 6-8

Prep Time: 5mins

Total Time: 3hours 5mins

Ingredients:

- 3 pounds of corned beef
- Cold water
- 2 bay leaves

- 6 peppercorns

Directions:

1. Put the beef in a large heavy casserole pot and completely cover with cold water. Next, add the bay leaves and peppercorns to the pot. Over a high heat bring the water to boiling point, cover with a lid, reduce the heat to a simmer and cook for between 2 ½ -3 hours.

Perfect Pizza

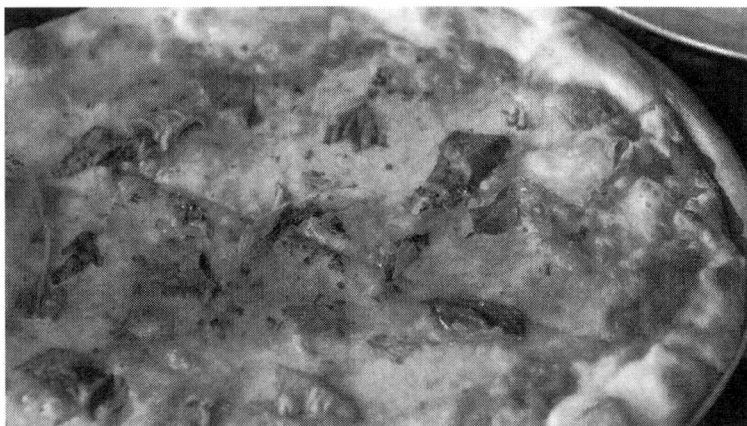

Just because you don't eat carbs doesn't mean you can't enjoy the delicious flavor of pizza.

Servings: 4

Prep Time: 15mins

Total Time: 35mins

Ingredients:

Crust

- 10 ounces of can chicken (zero carbs)
- 1 ounce of Parmesan (grated)
- 1 large egg
- Topping

- 2 cups of mozzarella cheese (shredded)
- 2 medium eggs (whisked)
- 1 tsp of oregano
- 1 tsp of basil

Directions:

To make the crust

1. First, drain the chicken. Removing as much moisture as is possible. Spread the drained chicken evenly on a rimless, silicon lined baking tray or sheet. Bake the chicken for 8-10 minutes at 350 degrees F. This will dry the meat out. Remove from the oven and transfer to a large bowl.

2. Increase the temperature of the oven to 500 degrees F.

3. Take the large bowl, add the Parmesan cheese and egg; stir thoroughly to combine.

4. Spoon the chicken-cheese mixture in a thin layer, onto a silicon lined, rimless baking tray or sheet. Lay greaseproof paper on top of the mixture. Cook the crust for 7-9 minutes.

5. Remove from the oven and add topping.

For the topping

1. Combine all the ingredients in a medium bowl. Stir well.

2. Spread the pizza toppings on top of the crust and bake for an additional 6-8 minutes.

Roasted Chicken

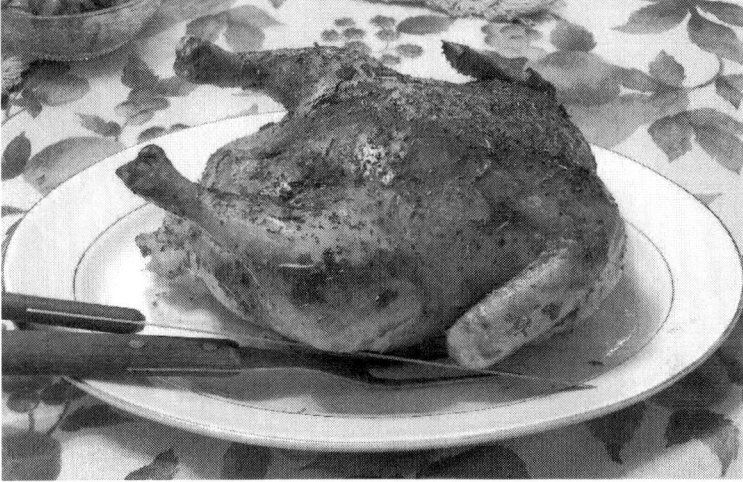

There is nothing more enticing than the smell of roasted chicken, to bring the family to the table.

Portions: 4-5

Prep Time: 5mins

Total Time: 1hour 30mins

Ingredients:

- 1 stick butter (softened)
- 1 (3-3 ½ pounds) whole chicken (thawed)
- Salt
- Black pepper
- Smoked paprika

Directions:

1. Preheat the main oven to 350 degrees F.

2. Gently rub butter all over the chicken. Place the bird in a roasting tin. Season well with salt, black pepper, and paprika. Cover with aluminum foil and roast for 1 hour 25 minutes. Remove the foil half way through cooking. (Based on a cooking time of 20 minutes per pound, plus an additional 15 minutes).

3. The chicken is cooked when its juice runs clear.

4. Remove the foil and serve.

Sesame Ginger Pork

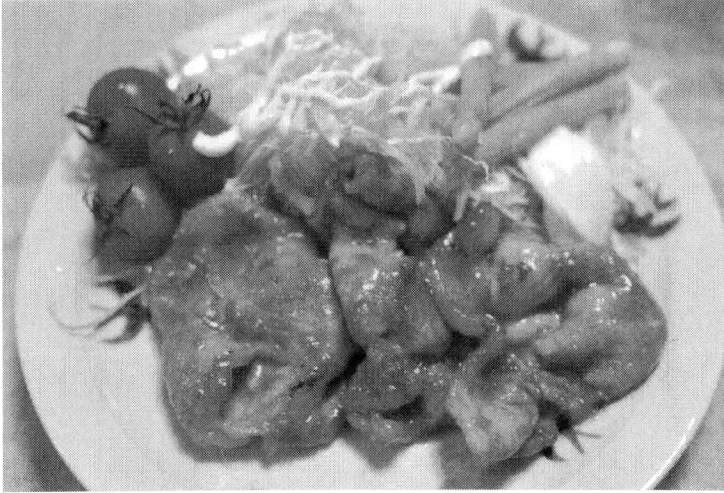

There are a lot of zero carb sauces and dressing in the stores at the moment. Check out what is available, they are great when roasting meat.

Portions: 5-6

Prep Time: 5mins

Total Time: 3hrs 5mins

Ingredients:

- 3 pounds pork roast
- ¼ cup of soy sauce
- ½ cup of sesame ginger dressing (zero carbs)
- Salt

- Black pepper

Directions:

1. Preheat the main oven to 350 degrees F. Put the pork roast in a large re-sealable cooking bag

2. In a small bowl add the remaining 4 ingredients and pour into the bag. Seal the bag. Massage well. Cut a few slits into the very top of the bag.

3. Cook in the preheated oven for 2½ - 3 ½ hours.

4. Take care when removing the bag from the oven.

Smoky BBQ Pork Chops

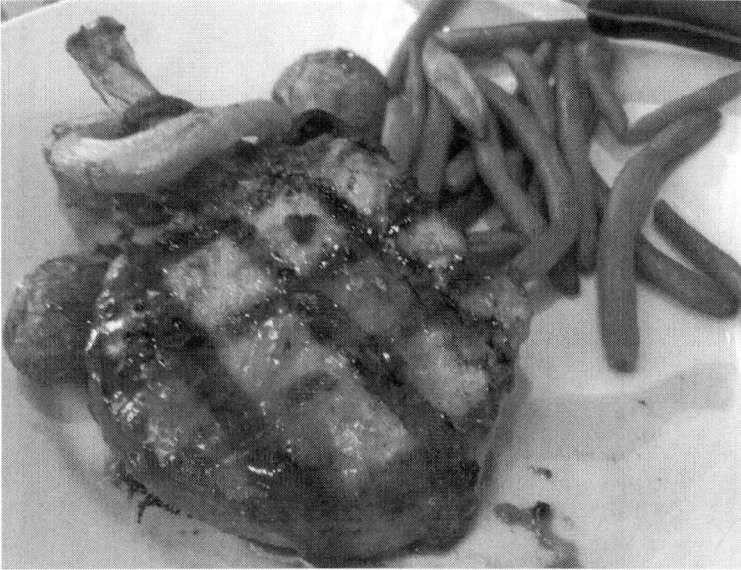

Meaty pork chops cooked in butter and barbecue sauce make a fabulous meal for an outdoor cookout.

Portions: 6

Prep Time: 5mins

Total Time: 1hour 5mins

Ingredients:

- 2 tbsp. of butter (melted)
- 6 pork chops (center cut)
- Salt

- Black pepper
- BBQ sauce (zero carbs)
- Liquid smoke sauce

Directions:

1. Preheat the main oven to 350 degrees F. Add the butter to a roasting pan. Season the pork chops with salt and black pepper and transfer to roasting pan. Turn the chops over so that the melted butter has evenly coated both sides.

2. Pour the zero carb BBQ store bought sauce over the chops. Sprinkle a little liquid smoke. Bake in the oven for 50-60 minutes.

Spicy Chicken Tenders

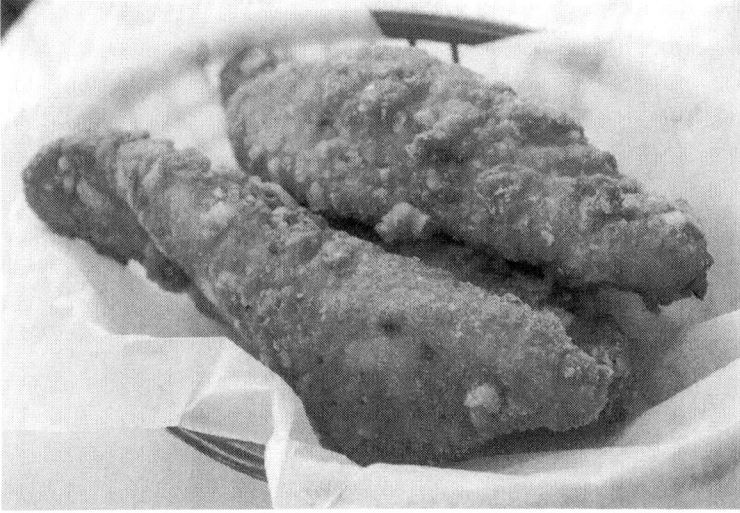

Cooking the chicken strips in peanut oil adds to the overall flavor.

Portions: 6-8

Prep Time: 10mins

Total Time: 30mins

Ingredients:

- 2 pounds chicken breast (cut into strips)
- 2 cups of crushed pork rinds
- Pinch of garlic powder
- Pinch of onion powder

- Pinch of paprika
- 1 tsp of cayenne pepper
- Salt
- Black pepper
- Peanut oil

Directions:

1. Put the chicken strips inside a re-sealable zip lock bag. In a medium bowl combine the crushed pork rinds, garlic and onion powder, paprika, cayenne pepper, salt and black pepper. Pour the mixture into the zip lock bag and massage to ensure that the chicken is well coated.

2. In a large saucepan, fry the peanut oil until hot. Remove the chicken strips from the bag and in batches, cook the chicken strips until golden brown. They are cooked when the juice runs clear.

Teriyaki Pork

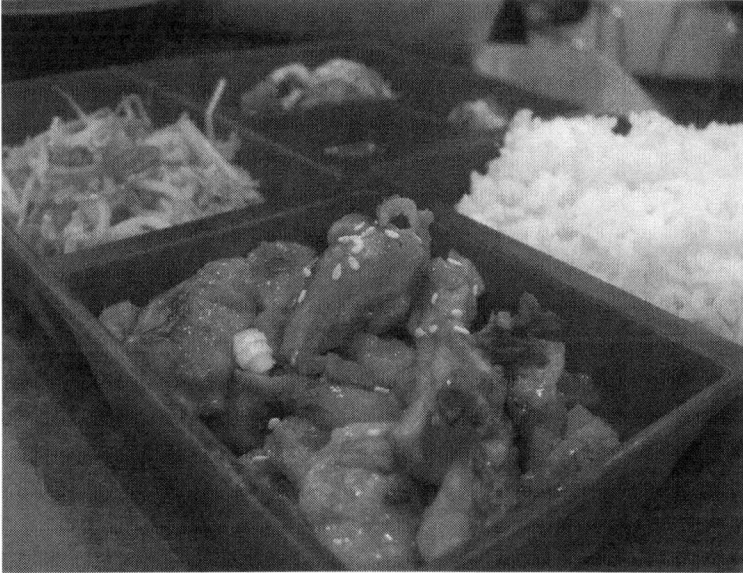

Peanut oil and soy sauce are perfect accompaniments to pork tenderloin.

Portions: 6-8

Prep Time: 10mins

Total Time: 8hours 30mins

Ingredients:

- 2 pork tenderloins
- ¼ cup of peanut oil
- ¼ cup of soy sauce (zero carbs)

- 2 tbsp. of rice vinegar (zero carbs)
- Pinch of garlic
- Pinch of ginger

Directions:

1. Place the pork tenderloins in a marinating dish. Using a blender of choice, blitz the remaining 5 ingredients until smooth. Pour the mixture over the pork tenderloins. Turn the tenderloins over to ensure coated on both sides, cover and marinate overnight. Turn the tenderloins a few times if possible.

2. Preheat the main oven to 475 degrees F. Line a baking tin with aluminum foil. Remove the tenderloins from the marinade and place the pork in the tin.

3. Cook in the preheated oven for 15-20 minutes. Turn over half way through cooking.

4. Remove from oven and enjoy.

Turkey Meatballs

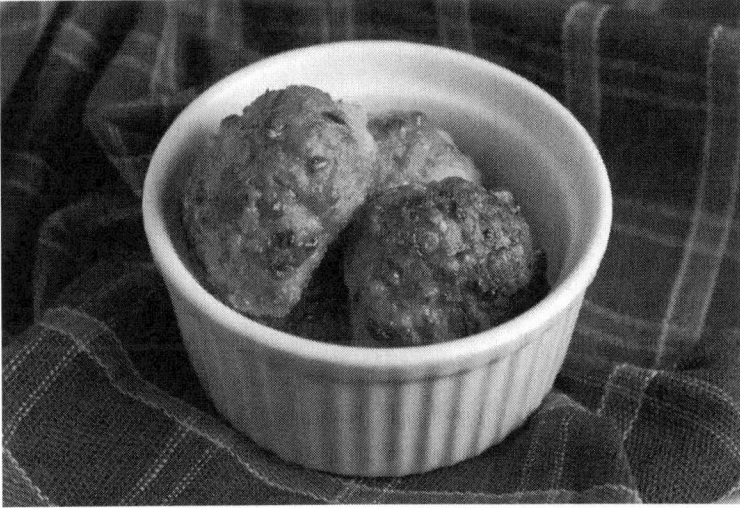

Turkey is a great alternative to red meat and pairs brilliantly with lots of zero carb sides.

Portions: 5

Prep time: 20mins

Total time: 40mins

Ingredients:

- ½ green pepper
- 3 mushrooms (remove stems)
- 1 cup of spinach
- ⅓ cup of Parmesan cheese (shredded)

- 2 eggs (beaten)
- 1 pound of extra lean ground turkey
- 1 tsp of parsley (dried)
- ⅓ tsp of oregano
- ¼ tsp of rosemary
- Olive oil

Directions:

1. Using a food processor chop the peppers, mushrooms, and spinach into small enough pieces that the meatballs bind together. When you have done this, transfer them to a large mixing bowl. Add the cheese and eggs to the vegetables and stir. Next, add the ground turkey and mix until combined. Add the parsley, oregano, and rosemary and gently mix.

2. Wearing disposable gloves, mold the mince mixture, taking a tablespoon at a time into balls of equal size.

3. Using a large skillet lightly coated with olive oil, place on high heat. When the oil is sufficiently hot, add the meatballs in batches, so they don't touch. Lower the heat to medium and cook for 3-5 minutes, until the meatballs are browned. Add a little more oil to the pan if needed.

4. Make sure you increase the heat every time you add a new batch. Repeat the cooking process until all of the meatballs have been cooked through.

Made in the USA
Middletown, DE
15 April 2018